T0208836

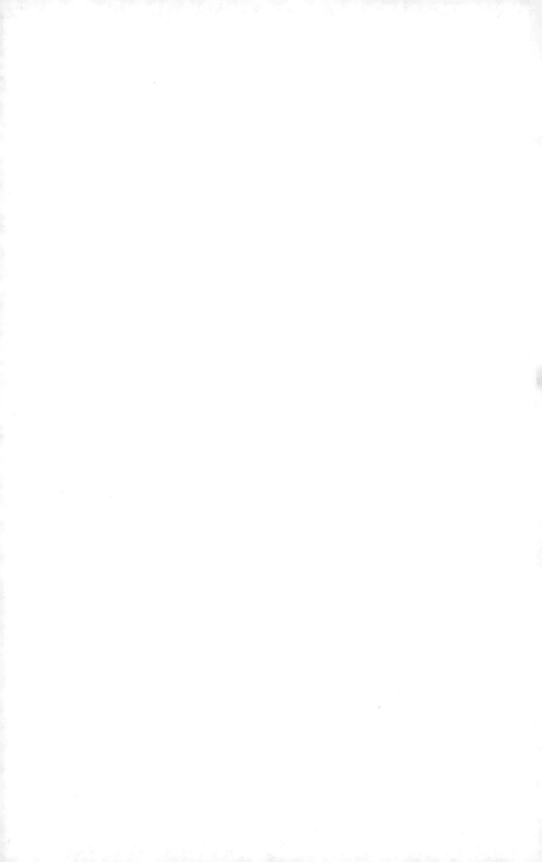

THE
FOOD
PARADOX

Eating More to Weigh Less

What is the Missing Ingredient?

ROGER L. WHITE MD

authorHOUSE®

AuthorHouse™
1663 Liberty Drive
Bloomington, IN 47403
www.authorhouse.com
Phone: 1 (800) 839-8640

Published by AuthorHouse 02/25/2019

ISBN: 978-1-7283-0186-0 (sc)
ISBN: 978-1-7283-0185-3 (e)

Library of Congress Control Number: 2019902278

Print information available on the last page.

This book is printed on acid-free paper.

What would you think if your doctor actually told you to eat more to lose weight? This is the main principle of the food paradox. Adapting its simple recommendations can add quality years to your life.

Doctors are often quick to prescribe medications but slow to talk about specifics of how to actually improve your diet and exercise. However, improving lifestyle is essential to reducing or avoiding medications and living healthier. This short presentation gives you practical advice on how to do this.

This monograph was developed from a series of educational lectures given to the employees at Organically Grown in Seattle, Portland, and Eugene.

I am thankful to the following people in making this book possible.

My wife, Emily Ann Rawlings-White, for teaching me much about nutrition and cooking.

My daughter, Natalie Reitman-White, for her inspiring work in the organic produce industry.

My brother, Howard White, for his lifelong support and encouragement.

Dr. Kenneth Cooper, founder of the Cooper Aerobics Fitness Center in Dallas, for more than fifty years of teaching about the health benefits of aerobic exercise.

And especially, my good friend Frank Tamru for his advice and editorial assistance.

If you were given the following choices, which would you choose

eat more, weigh less, and be healthy,

or,

eat less, weigh more, and be sick?

Clearly, most people would quickly choose the first option over the second because of all the obvious benefits. But how can one eat more and weigh less? This is truly a paradox.

Paradox is defined as a statement or proposition that seems self-contradictory or absurd, but in reality, expresses a possible truth. Paradoxes can teach us a lot because they get our attention. For example, they can help us look at old problems differently. In spite of medical advancements, obesity, diabetes, high blood pressure, cardiovascular disease, cancer, kidney failure, and dementia are increasing worldwide in epidemic proportions. Just giving more medications have not prevented or reduced these problems.

It is scientifically proven that eating more plant-based foods and becoming more physically active promote better health and longevity. To get more people to adapt to this lifestyle, understanding the food paradox can help instigate positive change.

These three components of the food paradox make adapting it successful.

1. Eat lots of low-caloric-dense natural—*real*—foods. Fill up with these foods first to satisfy hunger. At the same time, it is critical to reduce the amount of unnatural or processed high-caloric-dense—*fake*—foods that you eat.

2. Modify addictions to sugar, fat, and salt. Recognize your personal addictions. Limit these foods, and deal with psychological triggers for addictions.

3. Maintain regular, sustainable exercise. This is not an option. It is a necessity for good health. Dieting alone will not make you healthy or give you sustainable weight loss. To live optimally, you need endurance and muscle strength, which come only with regular exercise. Physical movement is also critical to making insulin in your body function better. How insulin works in the body is closely connected to metabolism and utilization of food. Without sustainable exercise, reaching your optimal weight and maintaining good health are almost impossible.

All of this sounds simple, and you have heard it all before. So if it is so simple, why do so many people choose a diet and lifestyle that cause suboptimal health instead of vibrant health?

Let's examine the above advice in more detail.

Food Caloric Density

"Caloric density" is a scientific term that means given the same quantity of foods, they will have a different number of calories. It is well known that foods, sauces, and drinks with more sugar and fat are higher-caloric-dense foods. Fruits and vegetables are generally low in sugar and fat, and high in water and fiber. These contents promote optimal digestion.

Fruits, vegetables, and grains are often called *natural foods* because they come from nature. They are also often called *whole foods* because they are less processed and have just the right combination of nutritious ingredients that no human-made food, supplement, or multivitamin can ever mimic. Humankind has evolved with plants. We need plants to survive. They give us oxygen and a sustainable source of food. Think of eating more plant-based, low-caloric-dense foods as being more in harmony with nature.

Traditionally, people who want to lose weight think in terms of eating less and exercising more. People often adopt gimmick diets to reduce fats and/or processed simple carbohydrates. This can be very helpful in improving health. However, people concentrate mostly on their new diets and make exercising a lower priority. However, dieting alone is rarely sustainable.

Initially, dieting alone can create a negative caloric balance and weight loss. The problem with negative caloric balance is that people are often hungry and feel deprived. Processed fats and sugars are everywhere and very tempting. Old eating habits quickly return—and so does the weight. This creates a feeling of guilt and a sense of failure.

The second problem to achieving optimal weight is the plateau effect. Eating less does not work in the long term because the body adapts to starvation by becoming more efficient at holding on to calories. The body also has a memory of its usual size and wants to maintain it. People find the plateau effect frustrating because what worked earlier to lose weight no longer works. This then creates the well-known yo-yo effect of repeating cycles of losing and gaining weight, which is frustrating and not healthy. Increasing metabolism with sustainable exercise is essential to minimizing the yo-yo effect.

Most people think of exercise as a separate activity from what they usually do. If there were a pill substitute for exercise, it would be the most popular pill ever. Our ancestors did not have problems with exercise because prior to technology, physical movement was needed just to survive. It was part of normal living.

Striking a balance between our busy but sedentary lifestyles and exercising becomes a real challenge. Exercise can take time away from what we like to do or have to do. Exercising soon becomes a lower priority. For some people, it can even feel like punishment.

Decreasing physical movement slows metabolism, which causes weight gain. Inactivity also decreases muscle mass. Muscles give both strength and the ability to burn calories. Loss of muscle mass is a common cause for weight gain as one gets older.

Sustainable exercise needs to be a habit, like brushing your teeth. Fat-burning aerobic exercise is necessary every day to maintain optimal weight. Some daily weight-bearing exercise is also needed at any age. These facts cannot be ignored.

Optimal weight does not necessarily mean being thin. It also changes with age. Optimal weight is intuitive rather than an absolute number. It does not have large fluctuations. At optimal weight, there is a healthy balance with your energy needs. You feel well, and you know it.

For good health, body mass index (BMI)—weight divided by height—should be less than thirty. Optimal percentage of body fat should be between fifteen and twenty-five. However, people should not be obsessed by numbers, a specific weight, rate of weight loss, or time frame to lose weight. Everyone is unique. In fact, I recommend that when adapting principles of the food paradox, one should not actually weigh himself or herself that frequently.

Obtaining fitness is much more important than any absolute weight goal. Here is another paradox. Someone who is classified as a bit overweight but fit can be much healthier than someone who is thin but unfit. Measure your progress by fitness rather than weight.

A mostly low-caloric-dense diet combined with exercise is natural. It is what healthy human beings have done for thousands of years. When you follow the guidelines of the food paradox, your body shape will change gradually over months. Be patient. If you have been in a condition of un-wellness for years, sustainable improvement will take months. But it will result in years of healthier living if maintained. Body acceptance and self-confidence will also improve over time. Optimal health is a lifelong goal, not an artificial weight goal.

Here are a few helpful guidelines and hints to develop your goals to eating more low-caloric-dense foods.

First and often forgotten is that your health begins with what you buy and bring into your kitchen. Think carefully about your choices, and take responsibility for those choices.

I find it helpful to think of a shopping cart as a large stomach. Imagine every item you put in your shopping cart becoming part of you. Then think of the health that you *want* to have instead of the food you immediately *desire*. Make your food choices be more in harmony with real food from nature rather than fake, processed food.

Instead of using a shopping cart, try using cloth shopping bags. Carrying groceries in reusable bags while you shop greatly enhances awareness of what you buy. You tend to make wiser food choices and do less impulse buying. More important, you also get some physical weight-bearing exercise. If you can't carry it, don't buy it.

To shop wisely, first fill your shopping bag 75 percent with low-caloric-dense foods like vegetables, fruits, whole grains, or potatoes (especially healthier sweet potatoes). A full shopping bag should be enough food for three to four days of meals for an adult. If you are shopping for more than one, bring more bags. And if you are shopping with children, make them carry their own bags. This can be educational; become a teacher of nutrition for your children. However, children learn more by example rather than what they are told.

Top off the remaining 25 percent of the shopping bag with small amounts of higher-caloric-dense foods as desired. For example, these items may include meat, fish, poultry, dairy, butter, tofu, eggs, nuts, and olive oil. When planning your meals, think of your high-caloric foods as complementing and adding taste to your low-caloric vegetables and grains rather than being the main course. An example is whole wheat pasta with steamed fresh vegetables. Serve with a fresh green salad with a little bit of balsamic vinegar, olive oil, and herbs and spices. This can be accented with small bits of broiled salmon if desired.

Look at your plate before you eat. Maintain the spatial distribution of 75 percent low-caloric-dense food to 25 percent higher-caloric-dense food. If you have second helpings, eat only low-caloric-dense foods. Even then, eat only until 80 percent full. There is a delay in appetite satiation, which is why it is best to stop eating before feeling 100 percent full. Pushing back from the table at 80 percent full avoids bloating and unnecessary calories.

Planning ahead is important before shopping. How are you going to eat the food you buy? Does it fit together to make tasty and easy-to-prepare meals? Avoid prepared frozen meals as they are highly processed. Learn to organize, and use your stock of food so that you always have the basics for multiple low-caloric-dense meals. Don't buy excessive vegetables, so you can use them while they are fresh. Shopping with a list rather than with desire makes this entire process much more efficient.

Before you go to the cashier, look inside your shopping once more. Ask yourself what foods are excessively high in salt, sugar, or fat. Return at least one of these items to the shelf. Stay disciplined.

People eat away from home more than ever in the history of humankind. It can be convenient and fun, but in general, it is high-caloric-dense and expensive. Staying on the 75 percent to 25 percent formula is much more challenging when you eat at restaurants, but it is not impossible. Be creative and assertive when ordering at a restaurant, and you can still get a tasty low-caloric-dense meal. One example is to ask for extra vegetables with a large salad with a small amount of olive oil and vinegar. Ask for the dressing on the side. A baked potato with mustard, chives, and herbs and spices can serve as an entrée and be tasty and filling. Another strategy is to share a main course to reduce intake of high-caloric-dense foods. Try to choose restaurants that are vegetable friendly. Avoid foods with heavy sauces and even vegetarian entrées with lots of cheese, which are high-caloric-dense. Ask for your food to be unsalted. Try to limit yourself to no more than two meals a week at any restaurants. This includes fast-food restaurants. Think more about eating and entertaining at home and more sack lunches.

Here are some practical recommendations to try to maintain the 75 percent to 25 percent ratio of low- to high-caloric-dense food when shopping. This is not an all-inclusive list but meant to encourage more learning.

The first thing you should strongly limit in your shopping bag if you want to lose weight is sweetened drinks. Probably the biggest offenders are soda drinks.

Consuming sodas is like eating processed sugar. The next time you order a soda to go with your meal at a restaurant, think of eating ten to fifteen packets of processed sugar instead. Sounds pretty disgusting, but that is really the amount of sugar you are actually consuming in that drink. These days, most sodas are sweetened with highly processed corn syrup, which is even sweeter than processed sugarcane. Corn syrup is also very disruptive to the sweet saturation center in the brain. This creates a problem of drinking these drinks to excess because there is less sweet satiation.

In addition to the obvious reduction in sodas, sweetened drinks of all kinds need to be reduced. This includes many energy drinks, sweetened ice tea, and even so-called natural fruit juices that often have lots of added artificial sugars. Carefully read the labels on these products for added sugar content, and think twice before putting them in your shopping bag.

Beware of drinks that have low-calorie artificial sweeteners. These ingredients can disrupt your neurochemistry. Surprisingly, most people who substitute artificial sweeteners for higher-calorie equivalents usually do not end up losing weight; they often gain weight.

Clearly, the best no-calorie drink is water. It is natural, and the biggest ingredient in our bodies. One of the best sources for purified water is eating fruits and vegetables full of natural water. Eating an apple or a juicy cucumber is like eating water. Stay well hydrated during the day with frequent sips of water. This reduces your appetite and makes you more alert. Dehydration causes hunger and fatigue.

What about alcohol? All wine, beer, and especially spirits are very high-caloric-dense foods. In excess, they all can cause significant physical problems. They all have risks for significant psychosocial problems. In most situations, responsible drinking causes minimal problems, but you should think twice before adding alcoholic drinks to your shopping bag, particularly if you want to lose weight. All alcohol promotes accumulation of body fat, particularly in the belly and hips. It is often difficult to remove because of alcohol-related insulin resistance.

Reduce the amount of high-dense-caloric fatty foods in your bag.

Meat, poultry, and fish can have a lot of nutritional value, but they all tend to be calorie dense. Preparing these foods in cooking oil and adding sweet sauces make them high-caloric-dense.

The same is true for dairy products. Cream, butter, and cheese are all very calorie dense. Lower-fat versions may not necessarily be all that low in calories because they have added sugars. For example, beware of added sugar in many yogurts with added fruits and honey. Coconut milk is also highly calorie dense.

If you choose to have cheese, remember it is a concentrated fat. Most cheese is also very high in salt, which can cause fluid retention, swollen ankles, and high blood pressure.

Dairy products can be not only calorie dense but can cause physical problems in people who are lactose intolerant or who have allergies and asthma.

A small amount of natural fat in the diet from dairy or meat can actually be helpful to curb appetite. They can supply minerals and vitamins that may be less prevalent in plant-based foods. However, it is extremely difficult to lose body fat if you eat excessive fat from animals or plants every day. Use fats only in small amounts to complement meals. A little bit goes a long way when using fat for flavoring.

Processed foods are altered from their natural conditions. This is why I call them fake foods. Most processed foods didn't exist a few hundred years ago. This is also true for processed white cane sugar, which we think of as so common today. Processed foods are unnatural and need to be markedly limited to obtain good health. If you choose a food that didn't exist four hundred years ago, hesitate before putting it in your shopping bag.

So how does a food become processed?

Fiber in fruit slows intestinal absorption of sugar. When you eat one natural orange, you get both the juice and the pulp, and natural sugar (fructose) is slowly absorbed into the body. However, if you squeeze several oranges and remove the fiber, the result is denser in calories than a single orange. Juice is quickly absorbed and highly glycemic, raising blood glucose rapidly.

Marmalade is highly processed. It is a little bit of orange with a lot of processed sugar that makes it high-caloric-dense. You lose almost all of the nutritional benefit of the fruit. Here again, a little bit of butter and marmalade on toast is rarely harmful, but a lot can be problematic if you are trying to lose weight. The calories from a couple pieces of toast with butter and jam can easily exceed several pieces of natural fruit or a handful of natural berries.

Highly processed foods are now very common. Most are high-caloric-dense and contain a lot of chemicals for added taste and preservation. Often, they don't even look all that dangerous. A few examples of these highly processed corn syrup–laden foods include most breakfast cereals, frozen pancakes, packaged bakery foods, cookies, crackers, and salad dressings. Freshly made oatmeal flavored with natural fruit, walnuts, and almond milk is a good low-caloric-dense alternative. You can also have oatmeal and fruit anytime of the day when you are rushed and don't know what to eat. It is much better than high-calorie salty pizza.

Many foods can be low-caloric-dense or high-caloric-dense depending on how you use them. A good example of this is the potato. If steamed or baked, a potato is nutritious and low-caloric-dense. As you add butter or cream, the potato meal becomes more calorie denser. Potato chips cooked in oil are high-caloric-dense. Traditional dips for potato chips are full of calories and salt. Rather than potato chips, baked potato wedges are good alternatives because they retain low-caloric-density and are filling. They can be used to accent salads or broiled vegetables. Potatoes combined with beans for protein make tasty low-caloric-dense meals. Low-fat yogurt and mustard are good substitutes for sour cream.

Adding steamed cabbage, green peppers, cauliflower, and other greens further enhances a baked potato. Another way to enhance the flavor of potatoes is to mash them with other steamed vegetables, like carrots or broccoli, and herbs or spices. Try steaming some yams or sweet potatoes and keeping them available in your refrigerator. They also make easily transportable foods for trips or long hikes.

Eggs are a good example of watching carefully the company your food keeps. A plain hard-boiled or poached egg is not all that fatty and can be a good source of nutrition. However, when you fry it or have it with cheese and bacon or creamy sauces, the egg meal becomes high-caloric-dense.

If you cook healthy chopped spinach with butter and cream, it becomes a high-caloric-dense fatty food with little nutritional benefit. The same is true when you add mayonnaise to salads and other foods. The salad become high-caloric-dense.

Brown rice with black beans and low-salt corn tortillas makes a quick, low-caloric-dense meal when you are hungry. Adding a little bit of avocado, tomatoes, grilled vegetables, celery, onion, salsa, and spices enhances taste and variation.

To curb the addiction to unnecessary snacks, have an abundant supply of fresh, whole apples, pears, or bananas always available. These can all be eaten in their natural state without processing or additives.

The following common situations can be real food traps for consuming undesirable foods.

Trendy coffee shops are everywhere. Gourmet coffee drinks contain lots of concentrated fat and sugar. Obviously, caffeine can be strongly addictive and triggers a desire for more sweets or creamy foods. A coffee break with a sweet treat can have as many or more calories than a healthy, plant-based meal. Drink coffee or tea without sugar or cream added. Decaffeinated drinks or plain hot water with lemon or sliced fresh ginger are good alternatives. Avoiding caffeine is particularly important if you have irregular heartbeats (atrial fibrillation) or high blood pressure. Caffeine commonly aggravates both of these problems. It is easier to stop caffeine rather than take medications with potential negative side effects.

Almost all foods sold at gasoline stations and convenience stores are highly processed. One should also totally avoid any foods from vending machines. These foods are not natural. Think of them as human animal traps, tempting but ultimately deadly.

Airplane food is generally high in salt, sugar, and fat. Alcohol makes this even worse. Eating and drinking these foods result in a flying hangover and swollen ankles. When you are tired, hungry, and bored it is a bad time to make food choices. But it is actually very easy to make your own food for a long airplane journey. I use an empty plastic container. I make a salad with steamed sliced potatoes, celery, cucumbers, tomatoes, herbs, walnuts, and a bit of yogurt. I seal it tightly so it does not leak. I also have steamed, mashed purple sweet potatoes with a little coconut milk as a dip for sliced sticks of zucchini. For dessert, I have some slices of fresh organic fruit. Passengers next to me often become very envious. I also drink a lot of water from my large refillable water bottle. This also ensures that I walk regularly to the toilet. Exercise and stretching are good during a flight. It also reduces the risk of developing fatal blood clots in the lungs. After a meal like this, I arrive at my destination feeling well with thin ankles.

Popcorn with butter and salt, candy, and refillable sodas at movie theaters are tasty but highly problematic. As an alternative, discretely bring pieces of freshly sliced apple sprinkled with cinnamon in a resealable bag in a purse. Just try to eat it quietly!

Protein-based foods are important in any diet because they provide essential amino acids, which are building blocks for cellular structure. Most people think of animal-based products such as meat and dairy as main sources of protein. However, eating low-caloric-dense plant-based foods like quinoa or lentils will provide necessary protein. Eating plant-based foods for protein is advantageous over animal-based high-caloric-dense foods if you want to lose weight. Plant-based foods usually do have lower amounts of protein than animal-based foods, but the human body does not utilize excessive protein. Even if you choose to eat animal-based foods, you don't actually need that much to fulfill your protein requirements. So just put less on your plate.

Not all plant-based foods are low-caloric-dense. But they can still be an important part of healthy diets.

Nuts and seeds are great plant-based sources of protein and fat. Although they are high-caloric-dense foods, they are natural and full of essential minerals and vitamins. They can be easily transported on trips. Get natural unsalted nuts that are fresh, and refrigerate in hot climates to avoid rancidity. Peanut butter and almond butter can supply concentrated protein and fat if desired after exercise and can replenish needed protein. Almond and other nut milks can be good alternatives to dairy.

Avocados and coconut milk are examples of how creamy tastes can be added to a variety of meals. Small amounts of fat from these foods may actually curb your appetite. But don't overdo it.

Green salads with vegetables are great low-caloric-dense foods. However, because of added oil, mayonnaise, cream, sugar, croutons, and other additives, they can quickly become high-caloric-dense. Even olive oil, which is often promoted for good health, can make a salad high-caloric-dense if used in excess. Keep the salad oil to a minimum. Try using oil alternatives to flavor salads, such as fresh herbs, lemon juice, apple cider vinegar, or balsamic vinegar. Even a few strawberries or blueberries can add a lot of flavor to an otherwise ordinary salad.

Every time you make a food choice, just do the math. It does not need to be an exact calorie count, but learn the mathematical principles of food caloric density. Use the 75 percent to 25 percent formula to fill up first on low-caloric-dense food. Most people will actually eat the same quantity of food each day. The goal of the food paradox is to fill up on low-caloric-dense food yet still have the same sense of fullness.

For thousands of years of humankind's existence, food has been challenging to get and often in short supply. The body needs carbohydrates, fats, proteins, salt, minerals, and vitamins to function normally. Our brains have been engineered to seek these foods that previously were sparse. Eating a large variety of seasonal foods is natural and healthy. However, now because of prosperity, availability, processing, and marketing, we have more of everything in our diets than ever. But feasting every day is not good for our health.

In reality, most foods are not good or bad. But when one combines continuous feasting with a sedentary lifestyle, poor health soon follows.

How did humankind get from eating to live to living to eat? The answer is simple—addiction.

The Neurochemistry of Addiction

Addiction is a very complex, mediated behavior that is triggered by a combination of psychological, sociological, genetic, and physical factors. Addictions are not signs of weakness. It is fair to say that everyone has some addictions. However, when they begin to adversely affect one's health, this is when understanding what fuels addictions is very important to controlling them. Everyone is prone to various food addictions. Understanding the role of the neurochemical dopamine in this process is helpful in making healthful food choices.

Dopamine, a neurotransmitter, is made in a small area deep within the brain called the basal ganglia. When released into the brain, it tends to give us energy and a feeling of well-being. Interestingly, dopamine secretion is increased during physical and sexual activity. The neurological responses associated with dopamine control reward-motivated behavior. This is a technical way of saying that if something feels good, we want more of it.

Narcotics, like codeine and morphine, are well-known, potentially addictive medications. Taken short term for pain relief, they can be wonderful in reducing pain and are not addictive. However, the longer one takes narcotics, the less effective they become. The first time one takes a narcotic for pain, dopamine is suddenly increased in the brain. The narcotic stimulates another natural neurotransmitter, endorphin, that also modifies our perception of pain and pleasure. However, when narcotics are used on a chronic basis, more and more of the drug is needed to get the same relief because dopamine does not respond as quickly. It becomes depleted. The feeling of optimism dissipates and is replaced by anxiety, depression, and a feeling of un-wellness.

Even if pain is not present, taking regular doses of narcotics is needed just to avoid the symptoms of withdrawal. Suddenly stopping a chronically used narcotic makes people sick. To prevent withdrawal symptoms, a natural balance of dopamine response needs to be restored. This takes time and is accomplished by gradually decreasing the amount of the narcotic that caused the addiction. However, even after the narcotic is completely stopped, the brain has a memory of the previous addiction, and it can quickly recur, especially during stressful times.

Addiction to alcohol is similar. Alcohol addiction is always more than just physical addiction. It has very strong psychosocial components. This is why twelve-step programs to reduce alcohol addiction stresses awareness of these psychosocial triggers. Some of the key components of the twelve-step programs are realizing one's problem is not unique, asking for help, recognizing self-worth, and helping others in order to actually help one's self.

Virtually all addictions have strong psychosocial components that maintain them. This is often the most difficult component of addiction to treat. Obtaining insight and behavior modification are extremely important to improving health. This is very true with the foods that we choose to eat.

Food triggers memories that make us seek out certain foods. This is particularly true of ethnic foods or treats that we may have grown up with. They often give us comfort beyond the food. This is not necessarily bad, but if you have excessive increased dopamine secretion due to sugar, fat, or salt, overeating soon follows. This leads to potential food addictions.

Anxiety and depression can play big roles in food addictions. If you are secretly eating high-caloric-dense foods when alone, this can be a sign of food addiction.

What makes food addictions more difficult to treat than narcotic or alcohol addiction is that you have to eat every day, and temptations are always there. Today there are so many bad but temporarily comforting food choices available. Chocolate seems to be everywhere when you have an addiction to it. And have you ever had a welcoming doughnut during a routine meeting or gathering? It's nice and given with good intentions. But the sugar and fat can be highly addictive because it strongly stimulates your dopamine center. This is also true for family dinners with yummy creamy sauces and extra-sweet desserts. Don't mix up food with love. It is okay to politely say no to foods that you know excessively stimulate your dopamine level.

Perhaps instead of putting so much emphasis on food for bonding and love, we just need to walk more together and talk. Some of my best conversations have been with people during long hikes. Movement itself can be very meditative and reduce stress and anxiety. It also releases healthy levels of dopamine. Perhaps this should be the first step toward behavior modification to reduce stress and anxiety when challenged by a food addiction.

Sugar, fat, and salt highly stimulate our taste buds, which in turn, increases dopamine secretion. But when constantly stimulated, this leads to dopamine depletion, just like in narcotic addiction. When this happens, you may robotically eat more sugar, fat, and salt to avoid withdrawal symptoms. Eating is no longer fun.

We erroneously start to think that we cannot live without our addictive foods. The solution is similar to treating withdrawal from drugs. The difference, however, is that completely stopping sugar, fat, or salt for a while is not physically dangerous. In extreme cases, supervised medical fasting may be helpful to curb salt, sugar, and fat addictions. There may be no physical withdrawal, but there is often significant psychological withdrawal. A break from these foods gives you time to recalibrate your taste buds, while at the same time, addressing the more difficult issues of psychosocial reason for food addiction. Addressing and gaining insight into these issues are not easy but critical to future healthy eating.

When trying to overcome a sugar, fat, or salt addiction, concentrate on changing your taste preferences to more natural fruits, vegetables, grains, and healthy herbs and spices. These foods are also delicious but in a different way. They do not have the concentration of artificial sugar, fat, and salt contained in many modern processed foods. Natural, real foods don't produce the immediate intensity of dopamine secretion that addictive foods do. These natural—or real foods—have interacted with our brains for survival for thousands of years. They are not the latest improved tasty treat from your fast-food restaurant that are designed to artificially stimulate your dopamine centers and makes you want more, more, and more.

Compare the difference in taste between a salty potato chip with a creamy dip to a slice of apple. The salty potato chip immediately releases a lot of dopamine in your brain. It is easy to eat a lot of chips and less apple. However, for better health, we should do the opposite. Even if you eat a whole bag of sliced apples, it would be much lower in calories than a handful of chips with dip. Also, with the apples slices you are getting a whole natural food with fiber and all the nutrition in the right amount. It is almost impossible to overdose on healthy foods. The more you eat, the more you thrive without addiction.

But this is easier said than done because addictions to sugar, fat, and salt are very powerful. Overcoming these addictions requires awareness. Perhaps a twelve-step program could also be very helpful for food addictions.

It usually takes about three months to recalibrate taste buds and reduce excessive dopamine stimulation in the brain. Being patient and concentrating on fitness rather than weight can be a good gimmick for transitioning to healthy eating. People who have strong addictions to sugar, fat, and salt need to make a conscious effort to limit these foods. In this way, these addictions are similar to alcohol addiction.

What about good addictions?

Good repetitive behaviors are sometimes called "good addictions." I am not sure that they are real addictions on a neurochemical basis, but if they improve health, I am all for nurturing them.

A good addiction is being prepared for situations that are challenging for you.

Have you every gazed with an empty stare into a full refrigerator and stood there thinking, *there is nothing here to eat?* You think nothing goes with anything else. Everything takes too long to prepare, and you just don't want to make the effort. You say to yourself, *I am tired and hungry right now.* To prepare for these moments of confusion, make low-caloric-dense foods that can be stored in the refrigerator for a couple days and used in a variety of ways. This is particularly important for busy people with little time to cook or those who have hungry children waiting for meals. This is very important in curbing food addictions. Having previously steamed potatoes or yams, brown rice and beans, fresh fruit, or ingredients for a nutritious salad always available is a good starting point. Also, avoid impulsive buying when shopping. This causes your refrigerator to have a lot of foods that do not go together for nutritious meals. Make a list of the basics that you need before you shop, and stick to it. Planning and preparation are very important to curbing addictive, mindless eating and gazing with an empty mind in front of an open refrigerator. Try to avoid this scenario. As a rule, you should never gaze into your refrigerator for more than five to ten seconds.

Exercise is another well-known good addiction. It not only improves healthy dopamine levels but is very important to proper functioning of insulin in your body.

Insulin Resistance: Today's Biggest Health Problem Worldwide

Insulin is a fascinating peptide hormone. It is secreted by the beta cells within the pancreas and is involved the regulation and functioning of glucose in the body. Glucose is the necessary sugar that the body uses for energy at the cellular level. It is essential for life. Think of glucose as the most important fuel that allows you to think and move.

The brain is particularly dependent on a regular supply of glucose to function. Without glucose, the brain goes suddenly into a coma. If not reversed, death occurs within minutes. Fortunately, we do not need to continuously eat foods with glucose or self-monitor our levels of glucose. Our body stores glucose in the form of glycogen in our livers. Through a series of complex biochemical reactions and monitoring, glucose is maintained in the blood plasma in a safe and efficient range. The only time we need to think about it is when we have either type 1 or type 2 diabetes, when normal insulin regulation is disrupted.

Insulin is highly involved in regulating the constant need for energy in the muscles, organs, and brain. However, today, with the foods we choose and a sedentary lifestyle, we get too much insulin in our bodies that does not function correctly. This is called insulin resistance, the hallmark of type 2 diabetes.

So how do we develop insulin resistance? Simply put, by eating too much of everything and being sedentary.

To understand this better, let's explore the functioning of insulin in type 1 and type 2 diabetes.

The discovery of the insulin hormone occurred in 1920. Researchers were looking for a cure for type 1 diabetes, which is the deficiency of insulin.

This occurs mostly in children. Basically, this is an autoimmune disease. Autoimmunity causes sudden destruction of beta cells in the pancreas. When beta cells are destroyed, insulin production is diminished. With diminished insulin, glucose metabolism is markedly altered.

Insulin acts at receptor sites on the surface of cells in the muscles and organs. Insulin is like a key that unlocks the receptor site. This is similar to how a key opens a door. When insulin opens the cellular receptor site, it allows glucose to enter cells, where it is used for energy production. If natural insulin is in short supply, the receptor sites remains locked (the door is closed). Glucose cannot enter the cells, energy production is depleted, and the cells become starved for energy. But at the same time, excessive glucose accumulates in the blood plasma. This causes multiple problems with hardening of the arteries (arteriosclerosis) and diminished nerve function (neuropathy).

When energy production is altered, the body looks for alternative sources of fuel. Fat is the most common alternative energy source to glucose. Fat is burned through a complex series of chemical interactions. This may sound good at first, but when it occurs over a period of time, the body develops ketoacidosis. In persons with type 1 diabetes, continuously burning fat significantly strains the body and cause a medical emergency and even death.

Prior to insulin therapy, patients with type 1 diabetes were actually extremely thin. It was called "wasting illness" and was fatal. Fortunately, now with insulin injections and pumps, relatively normal glucose metabolism is restored, and type 1 diabetics can lead a near-normal life. However, they are still prone to premature heart attacks, strokes, eye problems, and kidney damage. A prudent diet and regular exercise are very important in preventing these complications. Recently, it was found that regular exercise plays an even greater role than diet in preventing these complications.

Type 2 diabetes is a totally different process. In this type of diabetes, the body produces insulin, but it isn't used correctly (insulin resistance). Heredity, ethnicity, obesity, and advancing age can predispose people to this illness. It tends to affect mostly adults and gradually develops over time.

Insulin resistance develops insidiously without symptoms. In its early stages, it is called prediabetes. It may not even show up on many routine blood tests. Prediabetes is now epidemic in young adults and even children. With insulin resistance insulin that is made in the body does not interact appropriately with the cellular receptors. In other words, insulin is present but does not fully unlock the receptor sites on the cells. It is like the door is only partially open, and only small amounts of glucose can get into the cell. However, over time, higher levels of insulin are required to open the door (receptor site) to allow glucose to enter the cell. The beta cells in the pancreas are overstimulated to make more insulin to overcome the defect at the receptor sites. Blood glucose eventually becomes elevated and has the same adverse effects as seen in type 1 diabetes. Although medications can lower blood glucose, it is mostly regular aerobic exercise that will restore insulin's normal function at the receptor site. This limits the complications of diabetes *better* than medications alone. In addition, weight loss related to regular exercise further improves insulin sensitivity at the receptor sites. If you have diabetes do not rely on medications alone to prevent long term complications of diabetes.

Excess insulin also promotes abnormal storage of fat in the body. It acts like growth hormone to stimulate fat growth in the intra-abdominal tissues. Losing fat in these areas of the body is very challenging because excessive insulin is always stimulating intra-abdominal fat growth. A mildly fatty abdomen can be the first sign of prediabetes or type 2 diabetes. Interestingly, even people who are thin but do not exercise can also have harmful intra-abdominal fat. It is seen with computerized tomographic scans of the abdomen. Presence of intra-abdominal fat is a predictor of future heart attacks. But it can be mostly eliminated with regular aerobic exercise.

Excess insulin from type 2 diabetes also causes inflammation and toxicity to blood vessels. This causes diffuse premature arteriosclerosis. Not only are heart attacks, strokes, kidney failure, and dementia again increased, but the risks for infections and cancers are increased. These are all late manifestations of insulin resistance that has been going on often without symptoms for many years. Sudden death from cardiac arrhythmia from so-called silent heart attacks is often the first sign of insulin-resistant-associated coronary arteriosclerosis.

A plant-based diet with low-caloric-dense foods is excellent for the treatment of both types of diabetes. But here again the best diet alone will not control diabetes. Regular exercise is essential to preventing the long-term complications of diabetes.

Concentrate more on making your insulin receptor sites work better than just thinking about lowering your blood glucose level. Walking fifteen minutes after each meal helps this very much. Imagine a little bird on your shoulder every time you eat that says, "Walk, walk, walk."

WHAT ABOUT POPULAR, TRENDY DIETS?

People frequently talk about diets. There are numerous best-selling books that promote newer and better gimmicks. Here are a few comments related to some of these popular diets.

Are high-protein/low-carbohydrate diets effective for losing weight?

The simple answer is yes in the short term and probably no in the long term.

High-protein/low-carbohydrate diets function by trying to change the body's metabolism. More foods high in protein are eaten (mostly animal products) while eliminating most carbohydrates (especially refined sugar, bread, pasta, sugary drinks, and alcohol). The goal of the diet is to starve the body of carbohydrates and force the body to burn reserves of fat instead.

Burning fat is helpful for weight loss. As fat is burned, ketones are eliminated through the urine. Testing for ketones in the urine can be done to see if the diet is actually working and burning fat. People often like the high-protein diets because they are able to eat more meat, although totally restricting carbohydrates can be a challenge.

Paradoxically, starving the body of carbohydrates can actually mimic type 1 diabetes with ketoacidosis. Before synthetic insulin was available, most type 1 diabetics died of ketoacidosis. Fortunately, with insulin treatment, diabetic ketoacidosis is rare, and life-threatening ketoacidosis with high-protein diets is also rare.

In the short term, many people who are significantly overweight who eat high-protein/low-carbohydrate diets will lose weight and are delighted. Having some protein and fat in the diet also helps to satiate appetite. Satiation is a feeling of fullness, so you eat less. With some protein in the diet, people are less likely to eat between meals. All this sounds good. So, what is the problem?

The problem is that creating an artificial state of starvation is not healthy in most people. The body will adapt and try to change from what it perceives as a state of starvation. People will often then have a strong craving for foods that are high in carbohydrates. When giving in to temptation, they consume carbohydrates in excess, which causes weight gain. Weight fluctuates through the yo-yo effect.

People who succeed in long-term weight reduction with high-protein diets almost always increase their regular exercise and also eat moderate amounts of vegetables. They avoid sugary drinks and alcohol. They develop a healthy balance that is appropriate for their body types and metabolism. This is the main component of most paleo diets, which are modified high-protein/low-carbohydrate diets. They try to mimic diets of our very ancient ancestors, who were hunters and gatherers and not growing crops of carbohydrates (wheat, rice, and potatoes). But obviously, there have been lots of benefits for societies over the past several thousand years with farmed foods.

High-protein/low-carbohydrates diets can be very helpful in people who are markedly obese and have difficulty exercising. They can begin weight loss by gradually burning fat through changing their metabolism. With some fat loss small amounts of exercise become easier. Here again, the ultimate goal with chronic obesity should be improved fitness. It is fitness rather than just weight loss that reduces the complications of obesity the most. This is also true for people who have bariatric weight reduction surgery. Exercise is still the key component needed for improved long-term health.

The unanswered question with high-protein/low-carbohydrate diets is if chronic mild ketoacidosis in the body causes ill-health or even promotes cancer. Fortunately, ketoacidosis is probably not severe in most people on high-protein diets. However, in people with significant kidney disease, high-protein diets can cause severe acidosis and should be avoided.

Another potential adverse consequence of the high-protein diets is consuming excessive animal-based foods. This can adversely influence body cholesterol and cause cardiovascular illnesses. It is well documented that cardiovascular illness and cancer increase in societies as people eat more animal products. Also, raising animals instead of plants for food production is much more damaging to our environment and overall more expensive.

Again, numerous long-term studies have shown predominately plant-based diets significantly improve health over diets that depend on large amounts of animal products. If nothing else, plant-based diets tend to reduce indigestion, promote better bowel movements, lead to less irritable bowel illness, promote less body aches, decrease lethargy, and decrease ankle swelling. All great!

Vegan diets are totally plant based without any animal products. They have been recommended to slow or reverse the progression of cancer and heart disease, improve symptoms of multiple sclerosis, markedly reduce blood pressure, and reduce the risk of dementia, in addition to enhancing longevity. Even having just a few more vegetarian or vegan meals a week can improve your health and become a healthy habit. The most important thing is to find something that works for you, your lifestyle, and social situation.

Should people have fat in their diets?

Here again, the answer is both simple and complex. All fats are concentrated calories and, therefore, a prime cause of obesity. However, to have optimal growth and development as a child and maintain health as an adult, fats are needed in the diet. Plant-based fats, like olive oil, have been shown to be beneficial. This is an important component of the so-called Mediterranean diet, which has demonstrated reduction in cardiovascular disease, diabetes, dementia, and even erectile and sexual dysfunction. Diets that are higher in omega-three fatty acids (often found in fatty fish) demonstrate similar benefits. Omega-three fatty acids are also present in flax seeds and other plants. The important thing to remember is that there is no perfect diet for everyone. However, if you are trying to lose weight, added fats and refined sugar in the diet definitely need to be limited.

But what is the missing ingredient for a successful diet to improve your health?

If you have not already gotten the main message of this monograph, the most important recommendation for achieving better health is to concentrate first on fitness. This is the most important part of understanding the food paradox because the missing ingredient in any successful diet is not food but exercise.

As you can see, improving fitness not only enhances weight loss, it also curbs food addictions and is very important for reducing insulin resistance. Exercise is the magic ingredient that makes almost any diet work better and makes you healthier—regardless of your weight, body build, or age. Unfortunately, exercise is not a pill or a quick-fix that comes without effort. But the good health associated with exercise can also be a healthy addiction. After all, physical movement is what human beings have needed for thousands of years to survive. Is it no wonder that we have so many health problems when we suddenly reduce natural physical activity and adopt unnatural sedentary habits?

The relationship between exercise with good health is further strengthened by understanding the concept of sarcopenia.

"Sarcopenia" is the medical term for muscle loss. This is becoming our number-one health-related problem as people age. A sedentary lifestyle is also causing premature epidemic sarcopenia in young people. Sarcopenia causes disability, bone fractures, immobility, isolation, multiple illnesses, and premature death. With age and diminished hormones muscles atrophy; however, the biggest single cause of atrophy is inactivity. Muscle is replaced by fat and fibrous tissue. Having less muscle mass creates more fat. With increasing weight, people naturally feel less active and develop more sarcopenia. It becomes a vicious downward cycle of ill-health.

Yet, research is showing that sarcopenia is not inevitable with age. It is partially reversible at any age, but it is more challenging to reverse the older you are. Therefore, improving muscle function begins as a child, and maintaining it should be a lifelong process.

What is even more frightening is that sarcopenia can develop at any age, even in many people who exercise on a regular basis. This is because people are under-exercising and not really exercising their muscles enough on a regular basis. Muscles need periodic stressing (doing more than usual) to maintain optimal health. Just casually walking or doing water aerobics once a week is not enough to maintain and improve muscle mass and balance all the sitting that you do and time spent on the computer or watching television. You need to do something that is strenuous for your muscles every day. But not too much. Finding this zone can be a challenge and takes experimentation and experience. Some strenuous exercise needs to be part of any exercise program. Some muscle fatigue after exercise is a good thing. A lot of fatigue and soreness is not. Avoid injury.

Allowing adequate rest and recovery of muscles after exercise is very important. Good sleep is also important for good muscle recovery. Exercise itself enhances good sleep. Sometimes consulting an experienced personal trainer can give you new insight to find the zone for appropriate exercise that will give you the best results.

Achieving optimal weight with the right balance of muscle mass and conditioning is the best first step to any health-improvement program. This is literally the elephant in the room that must not be ignored. And clearly, most people are obese because they eat too much calorie-dense food—and less real food—combined with little or no exercise. Because it is so important, exercise is the great equalizer that makes almost any diet work. If you exercise on a regular basis, your body will find its own optimal weight and reduce sarcopenia.

Likewise, even the best plant-based diet will fail if regular exercise is not included. In other words, a sedentary vegetarian may not necessarily be healthier than a carnivore who vigorously exercises every day. The key of any lifestyle improvement program is to recognize individual triggers for addiction and to overcome laziness that modern conveniences have created.

Combining some weight-training exercise with adequate good-quality protein intake is important to preventing and reversing sarcopenia. This also reduces development of osteoporosis. Plant-based diets can contain adequate protein and minerals for good health. It just takes education.

Riding in a car is fast, comfortable, and efficient. However, it also promotes sarcopenia and is a disconnection from normal human movement. To prevent sarcopenia and reconnect to natural movement, try to do at least thirty minutes of extra walking exercise for every hour spent in the car. If you are frequently in a car for more than four hours a day, you may think this recommendation is impossible. However, you are at high risk for developing sarcopenia. If this is you, perhaps you should consult a physical trainer to bring balance into your life and preserve muscle health before it is too late. Also, if possible, bicycle to work or when shopping.

Every lifestyle improvement program that succeeds begins with planning, commitment, and discipline. Being aware of one's specific health needs and educating and adjusting as life changes are important.

As stated at the beginning of this monograph, you have a choice between good health and bad health. You can actually eat more high-quality, low-caloric-dense real food, exercise more, weigh less, and be healthier. But good health will not just happen without active involvement and setting priorities. Maybe after reading this, the first step is to take a walk for an hour and think about how you really want to be healthier. Do you want to be in the 20 percent who take control of their health or the 80 percent who just expect good health to happen without any work?

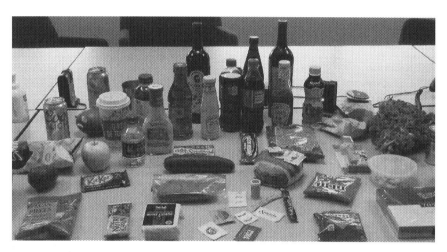

Every day, most people make about two hundred choices regarding the foods they eat, how they are prepared, and how much they eat. To lose weight, you need to choose more low-caloric-dense foods and less high-caloric-dense foods full of processed sugar, fat, and salt.

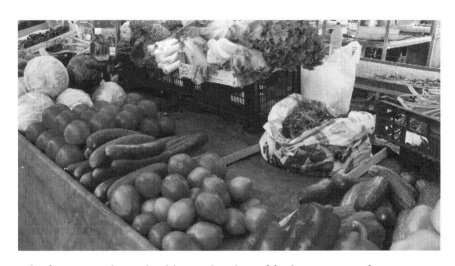

The first step to better health is to buy lots of fresh organic produce.

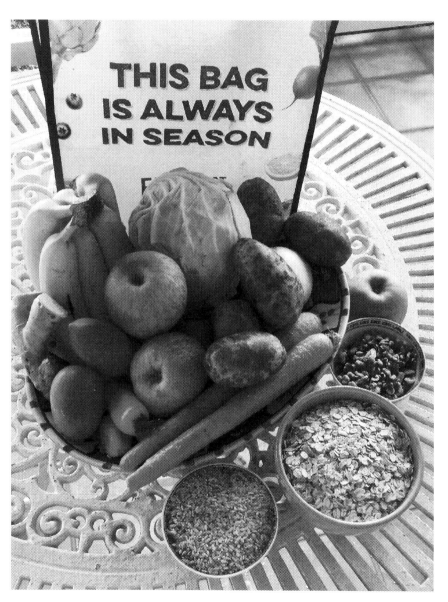

First, fill 75 percent of your shopping bag with low-caloric-dense food before buying anything else.

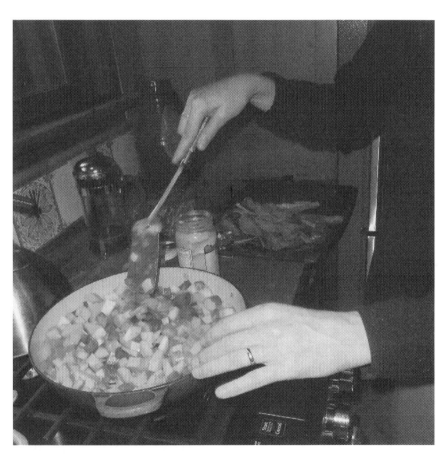

When preparing foods, minimize the use of cooking oils and processed sauces.

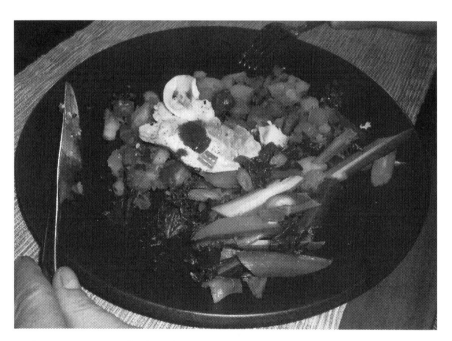

When serving your food, make sure that 75 percent of your plate is filled with low-caloric-dense food, and eat this first.

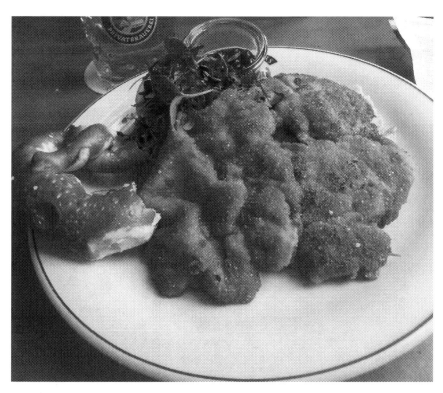

Although tasty, limit animal-based foods that are high-caloric-dense, particularly when cooked in oil. Fill up first with a fresh green salad with minimal salad dressing. Drink water instead of alcohol or sodas.

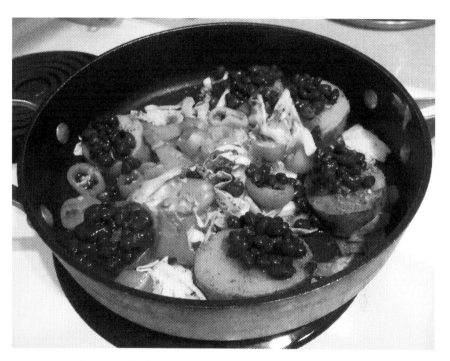

Eat more plant-based foods. Steaming potatoes with black beans, cooked onions, cabbage, peppers, spices, and a small amount of apple cider vinegar in a single pan can be quick and tasty. Stop eating when you are 80 percent full.

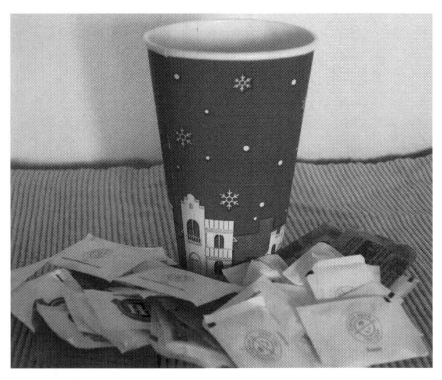

Avoid drinks with processed white sugar. For example, soda, many fruit juices, and energy drinks. Each of these drinks is equivalent to eating ten or more packets of processed white sugar. Yuck!

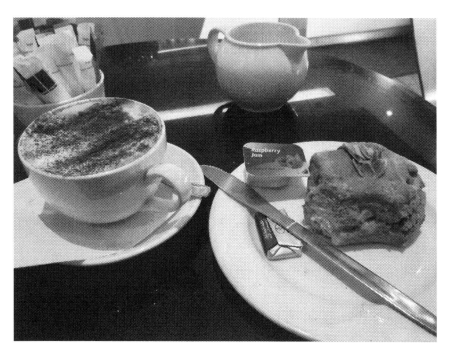

Beware of caloric-dense drinks full of fat and sugar in fancy coffee shops, particularly when combined with sugary treats. The amounts of calories consumed in a coffee break can be greater than a plate full of tasty vegetables and steamed potatoes with mustard.

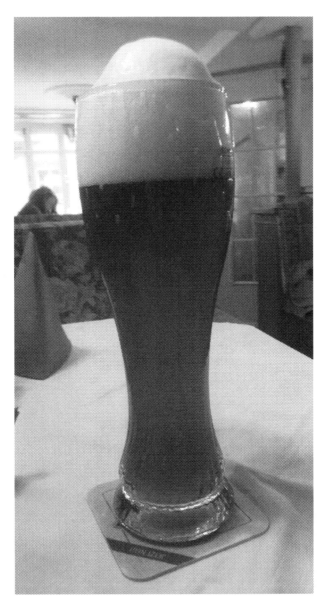

Beware of high-caloric-dense beer and wine. If you are trying to lose weight, they need to be markedly limited. They are also highly glycemic.

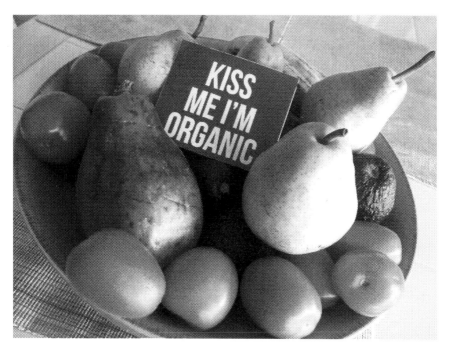

Base your meals and snacks around fresh organic produce. When you eat organic, you will kiss better. "Alles Liebe und Aloha-All Love and Aloha"

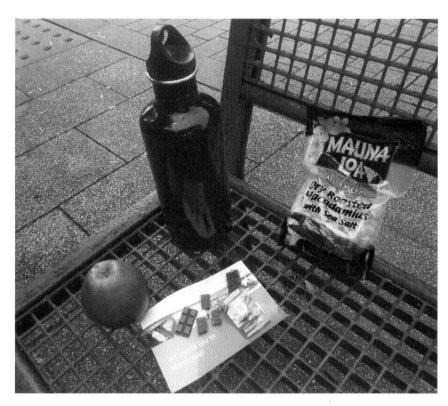

Always be prepared. Bring your own water in a bottle. Bring plenty of fresh fruit. Use small amounts of nuts to curb your appetite. Keep sweets to a minimum.

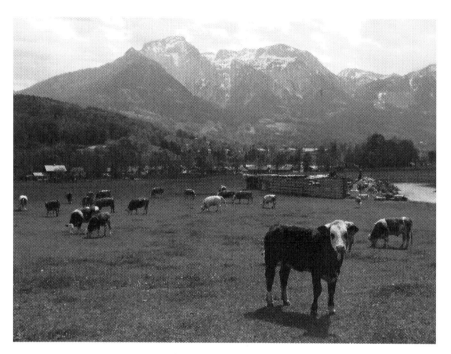

Mr. Cow says, "Eat more plant-based food. It is friendlier to the environment—and to me."

About the Author

Dr. Roger White is a retired clinical cardiologist.

He has been involved with emergency care, heart surgery, cardiac imaging, research, and teaching. He trained at the University of Chicago and has been on the staffs of Northwestern University Medical School and the University of Hawaii. He has published numerous scientific articles. He is a founding editor of the Asian Annals of Cardiovascular and Thoracic Surgery and the Journal of Preventive Cardiology. He has been a frequent lecturer in North America, Asia, and Europe. His main interest is in preventive medical care. He resides in Honolulu.

ADDITIONAL BOOKS BY DR. WHITE AVAILABLE THROUGH AUTHOR HOUSE AND AMAZON.COM INCLUDE

SOAR: Achieving Your Best Possible Health through Awareness, Author House, 2010.

SOAR: The Workbook, Author House, 2010.

Slimming with Daniel, More than a Diet, Author House, 2014.

Breathe: First Breath to Last Breath, Make Each Breath Count, Author House, 2016.